THE CUTTING EDGE

MEDICINE

Stem Cells, Genes, and Super-beams

Anne Rooney

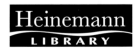

www.heinemann.co.uk/library
Visit our website to find out more information about **Heinemann Library** books.

To order:
☎ Phone 44 (0) 1865 888066
🖺 Send a fax to 44 (0) 1865 314091
🖥 Visit the Heinemann Bookshop at **www.heinemann.co.uk/library** to browse our catalogue and order online.

First published in Great Britain by Heinemann Library, Halley Court, Jordan Hill, Oxford OX2 8EJ, part of Harcourt Education.
Heinemann is a registered trademark of Harcourt Education Ltd.

Editorial: Sarah Shannon and Kate Bellamy
Design: Richard Parker and Tinstar Design www.tinstar.co.uk
Picture Research: Natalie Gray and Bea Ray
Production: Chloe Bloom

Originated Digital Imaging
Printed and bound in China by South China Printing Company

ISBN 0 431 13261 5   (hardback)
10 09 08 07 06
10 9 8 7 6 5 4 3 2 1

British Library Cataloguing in Publication Data
Rooney, Anne
Medicine (The Cutting Edge)
610
A full catalogue record for this book is available from the British Library.

Acknowledgements
The publishers would like to thank the following for permission to reproduce photographs: Bridgeman Art Library p. **5**; Corbis pp. **14, 16, 20, 24, 26, 27, 38, 49**; Getty pp. **7, 9, 31, 42**; Science Photo Library pp. **11, 21, 28, 33, 35, 41, 44, 47, 48, 51, 53**; Welcome pp. **4, 8, 12, 19, 23, 32, 37**;

Cover photograph of a digitally altered image of a person in a positron emission tomography scanner. A beam of light connects the person's head to the scanning equipment, reproduced with permission of Roger Ressmeyer/Corbis.

Our thanks to Ann Fullick for her assistance in the preparation of this book.

Contents

Any words appearing in the text in bold,
like this, are explained in the Glossary.

The big picture

Medicine – the science of healing the sick – has been practised for thousands of years. Even the earliest humans used plants as medicines and tried simple surgical procedures, such as putting splints on broken bones. But over the last 200 years we have made huge progress in medicine. We now use techniques our ancestors could never have imagined.

Hit and miss

Early medical discoveries came about by trial and error. From trying plants, fruits, and seeds, people have discovered some valuable medicines. Many of these are still used as ingredients in modern drugs. But in the process of discovery, many other people must have continued to suffer or even been poisoned. Nowadays, we test an idea for a new treatment in many ways before we try it on real patients.

Why didn't I think of that?

Some ideas are so obvious that everyone thinks of them. Most societies have developed ways of bandaging injuries and of holding the edges of wounds together. By watching the results of treatments, they have developed better ways of treating patients.

Some ideas come from nowhere, as flashes of inspiration. Other ideas build on existing knowledge. Often, combining knowledge from different areas can produce new and exciting ideas.

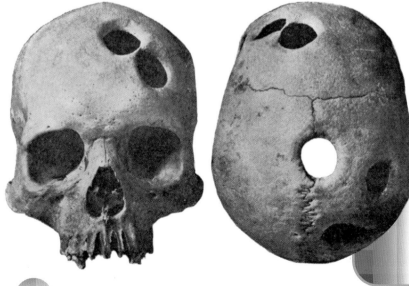

Early people in many parts of the world practised trepanning – boring holes in the skull to release pressure or "evil spirits". Evidence from bones shows many patients survived.

In many societies, it has been illegal to cut up dead bodies. The chance to learn how the body works from dissecting corpses led to major advances in medical knowledge.

Getting it right

Many years ago, a doctor who had a new idea for a treatment could just try it out on a patient – or even on himself. Now, there are strict controls to protect people from treatments that may turn out not to work or even to be dangerous.

Wherever it comes from, an idea is just the beginning. It must be turned into a real, practical application. Firstly, the idea, or theory, must be tested and often it is modified. In medicine, we have to be sure that new developments are safe, as well as make certain that they work properly.

The life story of an idea

A scientist developing a new treatment today often begins with **computer modelling** to see if the idea looks likely to work. This means using a computer to see how the treatment might work.

Next, trials on cells in a laboratory will test the idea further. If the laboratory trials go well, there is still a long way to go. The next stage is for drugs and techniques to be tested on animals to make sure they work. These tests check that the treatment does not do anything unexpected.

Trials on animals include giving too much of a drug or treatment or "overdosing" and combining it with other drugs or treatments to see if any problems are caused by them acting together.

Tests on people are called **clinical trials**. The new medicines are first tried on healthy people, and later on patients. Conditions are strictly controlled. The treated patients are compared with a **control group** of people who do not receive the treatment. Control groups are often given a **placebo**. This is something that seems the same as the medicine being tested, but actually has no effect (such as a sugar pill). The patients do not know whether they are getting the placebo or the treatment. Usually, even the medical staff do not know which patients are being given the treatment. This is so there is no chance of people's expectations affecting what happens to the patients. This type of test is called a "double blind" test.

If the tests show that the treatment works and that it does not have any unacceptable side effects, it can finally be used by doctors and hospitals. It can take more than ten years and cost hundreds of millions of dollars to bring one new medicine into use.

Moving on

For discovery to be possible, doctors and scientists must have open minds. They must be willing to challenge existing ideas and to try new explanations and theories. They must be ready to change their minds and to welcome new possibilities.

Is it right?

There are many debates about whether some medical treatments should be used and whether some types of research should be allowed.

Many people object to animals being used in testing, for example. Others question whether in clinical trials it is fair to give some people a placebo, instead of a treatment that might save their lives. Some people object to **fertility treatments** or **transplants** on religious grounds.

In many developed countries medical research is carefully considered by ethics committees. These are groups set up to discuss whether something is right or wrong. They decide individual cases, such as whether someone's treatment can be stopped if they wish to die. They also decide broader questions, such as whether to allow research using cells from human embryos.

Looking ahead

Progress has been very rapid in the last 100 years and the pace of change is speeding up. We are beginning to work with the individual cells that make up people's bodies, changing them to help prevent or cure illness. We are using the newest technology, including tiny robotic tools and beams of light, to look inside the body and carry out surgery. We can give people new body parts when their own bodies go wrong. But the diseases we are fighting against are changing, too. There are always new challenges and new areas to explore.

Adam Nash was specifically selected as an **embryo** because his blood cells best matched his sister, Molly's and therefore he could be a **donor** to save his sister's life. Some people feel that it is not morally right to select an embryo specifically in this way.

Stem cells

One of the newest and most exciting developments in modern medicine is **stem-cell** research. Soon we may be able to use these special cells to treat many conditions that are incurable today.

Back to basics

Stem cells are a special kind of cell found in human embryos and in some parts of the body. When a human egg is fertilized by a sperm, it divides rapidly, creating more and more cells. To start with, these cells are all the same. They are called stem cells. But soon the newly created cells start to differ. Some cells become the beginnings of bones, others the start of internal organs, muscle, or skin. We do not know exactly how the cells "decide" whether to become one thing or another. Understanding how they grow into different types of **tissue** could be the key to healing parts of the body damaged by injury or disease.

Some areas of the body can repair themselves by making more cells when they are needed. To do this, they keep a stock of stem cells. These are called adult stem cells.

At four days, a human embryo is just a group of cells, but the stem cells in this embryo can make all the other cells of a human body.

Landmarks in time

1950s First use of tissue from embryos in research: John Enders grows the polio **virus** in kidney tissue from an embryo

1956 First **bone-marrow** transplant (transplant of adult stem cells)

1973 First bone marrow transplant from an unrelated donor

Human stem cells were first grown in the laboratory in 1998 by two American researchers working separately – James Thomson and John Gearhart. Both believed that stem cells could help provide new cures for disease.

The first stage in developing treatments was making a supply of stem cells, which no one had managed to do before. Thomson's breakthrough came when he used a new **culture medium** to feed the cells. This simple change finally made it possible to grow stem cells outside the body.

How it works

Embryonic stem cells can come from spare fertilized human eggs left over from fertility treatments, or from aborted **foetuses**. They can also be created specially by fertilizing an egg or making a **clone** (see page 13). Thirty stem cells (from a single egg) can produce millions more over a few months. Many people disapprove of these methods for a variety of ethical and religious reasons (see Any questions on page 15).

Adult stem cells are taken from healthy, living donors. There is less debate about this than about using embryonic cells, as people freely give their own stem cells.

When stem cells are put into a patient's body, the hope is that they will make new cells of appropriate types. The type of cells made depends on where in the body the stem cells are put.

The first work on embryonic stem cells was carried out on mice.

1981 First removal of embryonic stem cells, from mouse embryos

1988 First treatment with umbilical cord blood

1995 Transplant of foetal brain cells from a pig improves the condition of a man with **Parkinson's Disease**

1998 Human embryonic stem cells grown in the laboratory

Ideas in action

We are just at the beginning of the work that can be done with stem cells. We can already use stem cells from within bones to cure blood disorders, and researchers are exploring many more treatments using stem cells. One hope is that stem cells could help victims of Parkinson's Disease, in which nerve and brain cells are damaged. The stem cells would be used to grow new nerve and brain tissue.

✂ Make the connection

Scientists have known for a hundred years that bone marrow produces new blood cells, though they did not know that it was stem cells at work. They tried to treat people with blood disorders by feeding them bone marrow. This did not work, as the stem cells in the marrow were not getting to the right place in the person's body. Stem cells needed to go into the patient's own bone marrow to create new, healthy blood cells.

Experiments on mice with faulty bone marrow showed that injecting marrow into the bloodstream could cure them. The first attempts at bone-marrow transplant in people failed because scientists did not know enough about the immune system. In 1958, French medical researcher Jean Dausset discovered how the body protects itself against foreign material. For transplants to work, the donor and patient must have matching blood types so that the body does not reject the new bone marrow.

Bare bones

Bone marrow is soft matter inside the bones. It contains stem cells that produce different types of blood cells.

Bone-marrow transplants were the first medical use of stem cells. They are now widely used to treat leukaemia and other disorders of the blood or **immune system**. Leukaemia is a cancer of the blood in which too many white blood cells are produced. Normally, white blood cells act to protect the body against infection and disease, but if too many are produced they clog up the bone marrow, stopping it from working properly. Sometimes a transplant of healthy bone marrow can help. Before the transplant, the patient's own blood-producing cells are killed with chemicals or **radiation**. Bone marrow from a donor is then injected into the patient. The new stem cells in the donated marrow take over, starting healthy production of blood cells.

When a bone-marrow transplant is successful, a child with leukaemia can be saved from death. Computerized registers of people around the world willing to give bone marrow are used to help match donors and people needing transplants.

New life from new babies

While a baby is growing in the womb, it is connected to the mother's body by the umbilical cord. This carries blood to the baby. At birth, the cord is cut. Blood taken from the umbilical cord contains stem cells that can be used to help people with blood disorders.

In some countries, parents of new babies can save their cord blood in case it is needed for future treatment. They can also donate it for treating other people.

Cord blood is put into the patient's bloodstream in a **transfusion**. The stem cells enter the bone marrow and enable the patient to make healthy blood cells.

Researchers are trying cord-blood transfusions for other diseases, including some in which the nerve cells stop working and muscles waste away. They hope the stem cells in the cord blood may be able to help the patient grow new nerve and muscle cells.

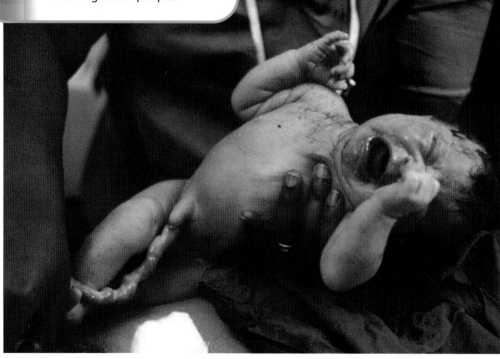

Designer donors

Sometimes, parents of a sick child have had another child specifically to use their cord blood. Eggs from the woman are fertilized outside her body, and then tested for how well they match the sick child. The egg that is the best match is put into her body to grow into a baby. Many people disapprove of this, saying that it is wrong to have a child chosen especially to be a cord-blood donor.

Super cells

There is a lot we do not understand about stem cells, but they hold great promise for the future.

In April 2004, scientists were surprised to find that damaged organs were improving and repairing themselves in children who had received cord blood. Stem cells had apparently travelled in their blood to other areas of the body and had grown new tissues. This was unexpected and will lead to new research.

Cloning

Cloning creates an exact copy of a plant or animal, or of some of its cells. In medicine, there are two types of cloning - reproductive cloning and therapeutic cloning.

Usually, a new animal is created when a female egg and a male sperm cell combine. It has some features from each parent. In reproductive cloning, a clone is made by removing the **nucleus** (centre) from an egg cell, and putting it into another cell. No sperm is used. The baby will be a perfect copy of the person or animal the cell nucleus was taken from. A whole new animal is made, which is a copy of its one parent.

Therapeutic cloning involves growing cells or part of an animal or person, which can then be used in medicine. The clone begins in the same way, with a cell nucleus being used to start a new embryo. But the embryo is not allowed to grow – instead, its cells are harvested and used to grow tissue.

Cloning landmarks	**1952** The first clone – tadpoles!	**1996** Dolly the sheep, the first mammal cloned from an adult cell, is born in Scotland	**2003** The first cloned male mammal, a mule, is born in the USA	**2004** Human clone grown to 100 cells in Korea; cloned bull created with cells from a bull that was itself a clone (serial cloning)

Copycats

Cloning has been explored first in areas of science other than medicine. It is possible that cloning could give us a way of producing food easily, or helping to boost endangered species. At the moment, it is still experimental. Most cloned animals die before they are born, or are abnormal. Scientists do not know why. They aim to find out by examining the clones that do not work.

It will be a long time before we know whether we can safely clone human tissue. Some groups already claim to have cloned babies, but none of them have been able to prove their claim. At the moment, cloning of humans and human tissue is banned in many countries.

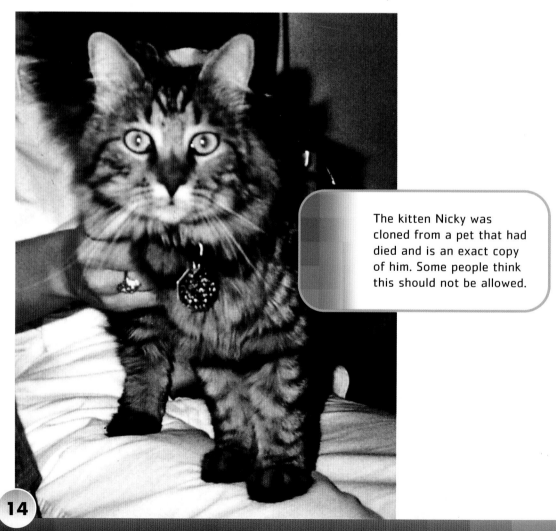

The kitten Nicky was cloned from a pet that had died and is an exact copy of him. Some people think this should not be allowed.

>> What is the future?

Cloning could offer a way of growing embryonic stem cells that match a living person. It means that people one day might be able to grow new healthy tissue from stem cells that are exactly like theirs. A clone could be made using a cell nucleus from a patient. Stem cells could then be taken from it to grow new skin for **grafts** or to make blood for transfusions, for example.

Any questions?

Stem-cell research is very controversial. Many people hold strong views about the issues surrounding it. These are some of the questions they raise and that you might like to think about:

- Is it right to use cells from "spare" embryos? (These embryos would not grow into babies if they were not used for research.)

- At what stage should a fertilized egg be treated as a person, with rights?

- Is it right to choose a child specifically so that its cord blood or other tissue can be used to cure another person? (These procedures do not harm or hurt the new baby.)

- Is it right or safe to create cloned embryos?

- Is it right to grow body tissues artificially?

Working with genes

Genes have been called the building blocks of life. Scientists hope we can also build new treatments and better lives with them.

Back to basics

All the characteristics that we are born with are coded in our bodies, in our genes. It is a bit like a recipe for a person. Genes are tiny pieces of information, held on **chromosomes**. A person has 23 pairs of chromosomes. There is a copy of them in almost every cell in the body. They are made from a chemical called **DNA**.

Through genes we inherit characteristics from our parents and ancestors. There are genes for physical traits, like eye colour and skin colour. Some genes might make us likely to develop certain diseases. Researchers hope that one day we may be able to cure some diseases by mending or replacing genes that have gone wrong.

Ideas in action

We are only just starting to apply what we know about human genes to medicine. As we learn more about how our genes work, that knowledge will revolutionize medical treatments.

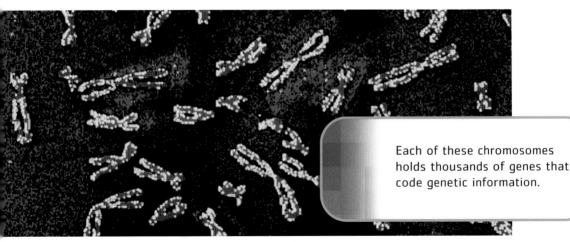

Each of these chromosomes holds thousands of genes that code genetic information.

Landmarks in time	**1850s** Gregor Mendel begins working on the principles of genetic inheritance	**1869** Johann Friedrich Miescher isolates the cell nucleus and finds it contains DNA	**1944** Oswald Avery shows that DNA carries instructions	**1953** Francis Crick and James Watson describe the chemical structure of DNA

✕ Make the connection

In the 1850s, the Austrian monk Gregor Mendel discovered from experiments breeding peas how some characteristics are inherited. He described how genes work, without knowing that they existed, and laid the foundations of modern **genetics**.

Later in the century, scientists saw chromosomes for the first time and realized that they are the key to inheritance; they also found DNA.

In 1953, with help from the work of Rosalind Franklin, chemists Francis Crick and James Watson worked out that DNA forms a double helix (two twined spirals). When cells divide, the double-helix shape splits and the halves complete themselves to make two copies. One copy goes into each new cell. This explained how **heredity** works.

Genetic screening

We can already screen people to see if they have the gene for some genetic disorders. These conditions are either inherited or caused by a mutated gene. (A **mutation** is a gene that has gone wrong while being copied to grow more cells.) Screening can be carried out before or after birth, and even in adults. Some kinds of very serious genetic disorder will become less common as screening prevents people being born with the gene and passing it on.

People who are at risk of passing on an inherited disorder, such as cystic fibrosis (CF), can have screening early in the pregnancy to see if the baby is affected. Some parents choose to abort a baby that is affected by a serious genetic disorder. Others continue with the pregnancy, but are prepared for the difficulties ahead. Screening means any treatment can begin as soon as the baby is born, giving it the best chance in life.

1972 Paul Berg snips out a bit of DNA and inserts it into another cell

1977 Researchers develop methods for working out the sequence of genes in DNA

1990 Start of the Human Genome Project to find the sequence of genes in all human chromosomes

2003 Human Genome Project publishes a full mapping of human chromosomes

Some people at risk of passing on a genetic disorder choose to have a baby using **IVF** treatment. In this, eggs from the mother are fertilized in a laboratory and checked for the defective genes. Only eggs that are not affected are put back into her body to grow.

Can we fix it?

It is a small step from discovering the gene that causes a disorder to wondering whether it can be mended. Knowing what genes do should make it possible at some point in the future to "fix" defective genes and help people with inherited diseases or disabilities. To test the theory that gene fixing could be made to work, scientists experimented on mice. They changed albino mouse skin cells from white to black. Albinos have no colouring in their cells. By repairing the gene that prevented the mice producing colouring, they made the mouse skin produce black colouring. An experiment on dogs has also worked. After more testing, scientists will be ready to try fixing genes in people.

✕ Make the connection

Cystic fibrosis (CF) is an inherited condition that causes mucus and fluid to build up in the lungs. People with CF need constant care and often die young. Screening for CF is possible because scientists have found out which gene has the mutation that causes the condition. They found it by comparing the DNA of healthy people with CF sufferers and carriers. It took a long time to find the one gene out of 25,000 that is different only in people with CF in their family history. The gene was identified in 1989 and screening started in 1990.

Police experts use DNA fingerprinting to help match criminals or the victims of crime to evidence such as hairs, blood, or skin cells.

>> What is the future?

The Human Genome Project began in 1990. Researchers in the UK, China, France, Germany, Japan, and the USA are working together to identify what all the human genes do in the body. We should then be able to build up a profile or full description of someone by looking at a sample of their DNA. Police forensic experts can already match DNA samples to suspects or victims of crime. One day, we may be able to give a full description of a criminal from their DNA, or tell before a child is born what it will look like or if it will have any genetic defects.

Making genes work for us

Work on genes and **genetic engineering** is not limited to people. Many medical benefits may come from working with the genes of other organisms.

People with **diabetes** cannot make the chemical **insulin**, which keeps the level of sugar in the blood stable. Many need to inject insulin every day. For years, insulin was taken from cows and pigs. In 1978, American Herbert Boyer put the bit of DNA that controls insulin production into a **bacterium**. The bacterium then made more insulin. Now, vats of bacteria produce human insulin for people with diabetes. Insulin was the first product of the **biotechnology** industry.

Mosquitoes carry and spread the disease malaria, which kills millions of people every year. Genetically engineered mosquitoes that cannot carry the disease may one day replace normal mosquitoes and help stop the spread of malaria.

>> What is the future?

Doctors hope that some forms of cancer may be cured by changing genes that have gone wrong in a particular part of the body. A cancer forms when cells reproduce too quickly, growing into a **tumour**. If the gene causing the growth could be "turned off" in the tumour, the cancer should stop growing. We need to find ways of turning the gene off.

Paul Berg, working in the USA in 1972, developed a technique called gene splicing. This involves putting a section of DNA from one cell into another. He used it to make bacteria cells produce proteins that they would not normally produce, making biotechnology possible. Much of the work in genetic engineering carried out today relies on this technique.

Any questions?

Changing the genes in unborn babies is a procedure many people are unhappy about, as it raises the possibility of "designer babies" – children designed to match their parents' idea of the perfect child. At the moment, scientists are considering only avoiding major deformities or serious disease. But the same techniques that allow us to do that could also allow people to choose other factors. It may be possible to choose a child with blue eyes, or who is intelligent or sporty.

Could genetic engineering or gene fixing be dangerous? We do not know the function of many genes, and do not understand how genes can work together. Changing genes could have some unforeseen effects.

Some people consider it wrong or dangerous to change the genetic make-up of other plants or animals for our own gains. Although we could benefit from improved nutrition or protection from disease, we might change the balance of the natural world in ways we have not considered.

All parents hope for happy, healthy children, but how far should we go to make sure that only "normal" children are born?

Man and machine

Science fiction is full of people with robotic parts. We do not yet have cyborgs – part person, part machine – but we are using more and more machinery to help in medical procedures and to improve the lives of people whose bodies are damaged.

Back to basics

People have used technical aids for centuries. Artificial limbs, spectacles, and old-fashioned ear trumpets are all old technologies for helping people with physical disabilities. Now we use far more advanced equipment, both inside and outside the body, to help people live with disease and disability.

We can now use **life-support systems** to keep people alive who in earlier times would have died. Life-support systems are complex technical systems that monitor and help regulate breathing, heartbeat, circulation, and temperature. Babies born before they have finished growing in the womb, and people who have suffered serious illnesses or accidents, may spend time on life support while their bodies develop or repair their systems.

✄ Make the connection

Heart surgery was made possible after the idea of chilling the body during surgery came to W. G. Bigelow in the middle of the night. In the 1940s he studied how groundhogs hibernate, then tried chilling dogs, and finally moved on to humans. His technique meant that five to six minutes of heart surgery became possible. Nowadays, heart operations can continue for hours, with the patient's body chilled to 12 °C (55 °F).

Landmarks in time	**1953** First heart-and-lung machine, which takes over pumping the blood and adding oxygen to it during operations on the heart	**1960** First **pacemakers** to regulate heartbeat	**1960s** Successful hip-replacement surgery

Here and now

A modern hospital is full of machinery and computers. To help diagnose conditions, doctors use all kinds of technology to look at the insides of patients' bodies (see *Super-beams*, page 30). Some patients use technology at home, or have little machines in their bodies that keep them fit and active. For example, people with diabetes can use a microchip tester to check the level of sugar in their blood. Some pacemakers can store information about how the patient's heart has acted.

We use many types of implants – pieces of equipment that are put permanently inside a patient's body. These range from quite large mechanical items like replacement joints, to very tiny electrical components or microchips.

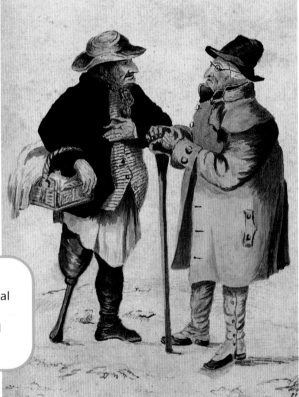

Early artificial limbs were crude. Now medical aids can perform many of the functions of real body parts.

2000 A robotic arm is moved by signals picked up from a monkey's brain and sent over the internet

2001 Microchips inserted in the eye to restore vision to three blind people

2004 Two disabled people succeed in controlling a computer using only brainwaves, picked up by a special cap

Ideas in action

Mechanical aids are becoming more sophisticated, and more computer technology is being used to help patients lead normal, healthy lives.

Beating hearts

Millions of people around the world are kept alive by pacemakers implanted in their chests.

A pacemaker keeps the heartbeat of a patient steady. It sends a small electrical charge to the heart to make the muscle contract and squeeze out blood. Early pacemakers were outside the body, attached to the heart by wires. Patients could not live normal lives as they were attached to the machine.

A modern pacemaker is fitted inside the patient's chest, so it shows up on an X-ray.

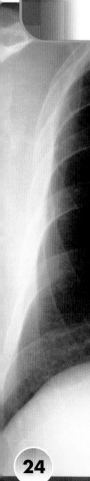

American Wilson Greatbatch was making electrical circuits to record patients' heartbeats in 1956 when he accidentally put the wrong resistor in his circuit. To his surprise, he found it pulsed and paused in the same rhythm as a human heart. He realized he could use it to drive an unhealthy heart. He showed his circuit to a surgeon, and three weeks later they connected a **prototype** pacemaker to the heart of a dog. It worked for four hours until it was stopped by body fluids leaking into it. Greatbatch spent a year experimenting with different ways of making and sealing the pacemaker. The first pacemakers were fitted to human patients in 1960. Pacemakers were the first pieces of electrical equipment fitted inside the human body.

Bioresponse

Early pacemakers worked all the time, whether or not the heart needed help. Normally, our hearts beat faster or slower depending on what we are doing. The newest pacemakers respond to the needs of the patient's body, helping the heart when it needs it but leaving the heart to beat normally when it does not. This type of system, which responds to messages from the body, is called a bioresponse system. Bioresponse systems in medical implants depend on computer chips. These track nerve impulses, muscle movements, and conditions in the body such as temperature, blood pressure, and levels of hormones (chemicals the body uses to carry messages).

>> What is the future?

Genetic engineering and stem-cell research may make even the most advanced pacemakers a thing of the past. Research on guinea pigs suggests that genetically engineered heart cells could be implanted to help restore a patient's natural heartbeat, making a pacemaker unnecessary.

Helping hand

For thousands of years, people who have lost limbs through injury or disease have used artificial limbs. Long ago, these were simple wooden peg legs, or iron hooks to replace hands. Now people are fitted with realistic-looking limbs made of plastic. Many of these limbs have myoelectric control. This means that electrical pulses from the person's nerves are picked up by sensors in the limb and used to move it.

In the USA, researchers are experimenting with implants in the brain stem to restore hearing to people with damaged nerves. The first hearing implants were tested in human patients in 2004. Implants in another part of the brain could restore vision. They have tiny photosensitive cells that respond to light and send an electrical signal to the brain, just like the cells in an eye working normally.

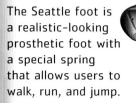

The Seattle foot is a realistic-looking prosthetic foot with a special spring that allows users to walk, run, and jump.

>> What is the future?

Scientists are working on ways of helping people to move an artificial limb by thought, just as we move a real limb. Researchers in the USA are experimenting with picking up signals from a monkey's brain. The monkey has its arm restrained, and is trained to try to move a ball, though it cannot actually touch it. Soon, it is able to use its brain signals to control the ball. As the monkey tries to move its arm, the signal from the brain is picked up and used to control technology to move the ball.

Another group has found that people can control a cursor on a computer screen using only thought. They wear a special cap that picks up electrical signals from their brains and sends them to the computer.

Scientists hope they can develop systems like these to help people control artificial limbs.

Microsurgeons

Could we soon have robot surgeons carrying out operations? Already doctors use an increasing amount of technology in the operating theatre.

Keyhole surgery (or laparoscopic surgery) involves making a very small hole in a person's body, through which surgery is carried out. Surgeons use a thin glass fibre with a camera on the end to see inside the body. They use microscopes attached to cameras to show an enlarged view of what is happening inside the patient's body during an operation. Some surgical tools are controlled by computer. They can be controlled precisely, which a hand-held instrument cannot be. Surgeons are experimenting with tubes less than a third of a millimetre across and knife blades a hundredth of a millimetre thick so that they can operate accurately at a very small scale.

Using the da Vinci robotic surgical system, a surgeon uses a screen and controls to work robotic tools that carry out the operation.

While the surgeon works with computers, microscopes, and robotic instruments, the patient's body systems are monitored, and **anaesthetics** are controlled by computers. Any change in the patient's heartbeat, breathing, body temperature, or brain function can be picked up instantly, alerting the surgeon to any danger or complications.

In 2004, surgeons successfully performed an operation on a dummy in a submarine, controlling robotic tools by radio while they were many miles away. NASA hopes to use the same technology to operate on astronauts injured in space.

>> What is the future?

The possibilities of **nanotechnology** – technology at minute scales –
are being explored in medicine. We may one day be able to send
microscopic robots into people's bodies to carry out repairs. One
possibility is that they will patrol the blood vessels, removing any
build-up of fat or looking for and destroying cancer cells. Nanobots
(tiny robots) would probably work with the body's chemistry rather
than use mechanical tools.

Any questions?

The most ambitious developments
in medical technology raise issues
of safety. The possibility of brain
damage from implants in the brain
is very serious, so research is slow
and very careful.

Life-support systems have become
so sophisticated that we are able
to keep people alive who have
suffered terrible injury and would
normally die. This can lead to new
and difficult questions about how
long they should be kept alive,
who should be allowed to turn off
a life-support system, and when
and how we decide when
someone is truly dead.

We have looked at technologies
that give people more control over
their own bodies. The flipside of

this research is the existence of
systems that control people's
bodies, and which could perhaps
be adapted to control them against
their will or in ways that some
people might think wrong.

Researchers working with rats and
eels have found ways of
controlling their bodies using
electrical impulses and ways of
teaching them new behaviour by
artificially producing pleasurable
feelings. Could these techniques
be used to create cyborgs – people
who are part human, part
machine? Or could we enhance
human capabilities with robotic
parts, giving supersensitive vision
or hearing, or great strength? Some
people fear developments like this
could be put to immoral uses.

Super-beams

Until nearly 1900, the only way we could see inside someone's body was to cut it open. Now we have many ways of seeing what is happening that do not involve any pain or risk to the patient. We use a variety of beams, such as light, sound, and X-rays to "see" inside the body and even to help heal it.

Back to basics

The light we can see and the range of sounds we can hear represent only a small proportion of the waves and rays of energy around us. With the help of computers, many kinds of rays and beams of energy can be used to make images that show us what is inside solid objects. We use lots of these in medicine.

Higher intensities of some beams can be used to make changes in the body and so can be used in treatments. Lasers, which are very high-powered and focused light beams, can be used like surgical knives. Radiation, which is energy emitted by atoms, can be used to treat cancer.

How it works

Images are made by measuring the energy that is absorbed or bounced back from objects. An **ultrasound** image, for example, is made by measuring how much of a very high-pitched sound wave bounces back as an echo. Some body tissues are more dense than others, so tissues give different echoes. An image is drawn by a computer measuring the echo.

X-rays are absorbed by some parts of the body and pass through others. This means they cast a "shadow" of the denser parts, which makes an image on a photographic plate.

PET stands for positron emission tomography. A patient is given sugar mixed with a substance that gives out tiny positive electrical charges called positrons. Measuring the positron levels in different areas of the body shows where the sugar is being used. The measurements are turned into an image by a computer. Tumours use sugar more quickly than healthy areas of the body, so they show up clearly.

Landmarks in time

1895 Discovery of X-rays by Wilhelm Röntgen	**1898** Discovery of radioactivity by Henri Becquerel	**1899** Radiation first used as a medical cure	**1917** Einstein suggests the possibility of lasers

Here and now

Different kinds of super-beams are now used both to treat people and to diagnose medical problems.

Radiation is commonly used to treat cancer. **Radioactive** matter sends out energy that can kill cells or prevent them dividing. The radiation is directed carefully at the cancer cells, though normal cells in the area are affected.

X-rays, ultrasound, PET scans, and other scans such as **CT scans** and **MRI scans** (see pages 33 and 36) are used to look inside the body and help to identify problems. While X-rays show up the bones, the others can reveal problems in soft tissues such as the heart, lungs, or gut.

> Ultrasound was first developed to help navigation at sea after the sinking of the *Titanic* in 1912. Now it is used to scan unborn babies to make sure they are healthy, and to look at organs inside the body.

YNRNG
58 db
5CU76
EPTH
34 MM
UTPUT
5%
FPS
20
EJECT
1
EDGE
1
GRAY
3
MOOTH
3

1950s Development of nuclear medicine, involving giving patients a mildly radioactive drink and tracing its route through the body

1960 T. H. Maiman makes the first laser

1972 Invention of CT scans by Godfrey Hounsfield

1988 First laser eye surgery carried out in Germany

Ideas in action

Over time, we have found more and more ways of using beams of energy to help us look at and heal people's bodies. The very first to be used were X-rays and radiation. As our understanding of these has increased, we have been able to do more and more with them.

From X-ray to CT scan

X-rays produce an image because they pass through most of the body but not the bones, which cast a shadow.

The first X-ray photograph ever taken shows the bones of Röntgen's wife's hand. Her wedding ring is clearly visible.

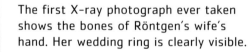

✕ Make the connection

Wilhelm Röntgen was experimenting with electricity when he inadvertently produced X-rays in 1895. He found that a **fluorescent** screen glowed when an electron beam was turned on, even though the beam was shielded by black card. He tried putting things between the beam and the screen, and when he put his hand between, he saw the outline of his bones projected on the screen.

Röntgen investigated X-rays thoroughly and quickly saw their possible uses in medicine. The first X-ray photograph ever taken was of his wife's hand.

X-rays immediately captured the popular imagination. People wanted X-rays of themselves, and X-ray photos of objects became popular curiosities. Doctors started to use them to look at patients' bones the year after Röntgen's discovery.

A CT (Computed Tomography) scan uses weak X-rays to show what is inside the body. The scanner moves along the patient, making a set of images like "slices" through the body. It sends the readings to a computer, which builds up a full 3-D model of the inside of the body. This shows all the organs and soft tissues.

The mathematics used to make the image from the X-ray information given by the CT scan was developed in 1917, but the calculations are so complex they can only be carried out with modern computers.

Radiation

Radiation therapy is used to treat many cancer patients. It works by killing cancer cells. But radiation can also damage healthy cells; people having radiation therapy are often sick and lose their hair. Scientists are looking for ways of targeting just the cancer cells.

During a CT scan, the patient passes through a circular machine that moves along the body, directing beams at it from all angles.

Radiation can be given externally, as a beam directed at the area where the cancer is growing. Or patients may have radioactive pellets implanted in their bodies to give out radiation where it is needed. The level of radiation is lower and it is kept close to the cancer.

The latest developments include using different types of X-rays. Some of these can be specially adapted to destroy only the cells in the **cancerous** tumour and leave other cells unharmed. This would mean fewer **side effects** for patients, as well as more effective treatment.

Cutting edge of light

A laser is a very narrow beam of light of one colour. It contains such intense energy that it can be used to cut through solid objects. Lasers were first used in the manufacturing industry to cut accurately. The possible medical uses soon became clear. Very precise cuts can be made, without putting pressure on surrounding tissue. Because lasers burn rather than cut, wounds are immediately **cauterized**, preventing bleeding.

>< Make the connection

The French scientist Henri Becquerel was interested in Röntgen's work on X-rays. One day in 1896 it was too cloudy for him to use the Sun as a source of energy for his experiments, so he put his photographic plates away in a drawer with, coincidentally, some crystals containing uranium. When he took the plates out, he found images on them caused by radiation from the uranium.

Becquerel did not explore radiation further, but Marie Curie and her husband Pierre, devoted their lives to working on it. They discovered other sources of radiation and found out that radiation decays over time. This property makes it useful in **diagnostic** medicine.

Radiation was first used as a medical cure in 1899. But it was not until physicists found out more about the atom that the full potential for using radiation in medicine became clear.

One of the first medical uses of lasers was for eye surgery. Lasers are used to cut away tiny amounts of tissue from the eye, reshaping it to correct vision problems.

The lasers are so accurate that they can cut to within one millionth of an inch.

Lasers featured as weapons in science-fiction stories for years before becoming a reality in 1960. Now we use them for surgery, but not yet as weapons.

Lasers can also be used to cure bad breath, killing the bacteria that cause it and sealing the areas where they live on the tonsils.

Magic with magnets

Magnetic resonance imaging, or MRI, uses a magnetic field to build up a 2-D image or 3-D model of the inside of the body.

The main magnet in an MRI scanner is very strong (around 20,000 times stronger than the Earth's magnetic field). However, applying even strong magnetism to the body is not thought to be harmful. The MRI scanner works by measuring how quickly parts of the body return to normal after a magnetic field is applied. The scanner measures energy from the body and turns it into an image.

MRI depends on detailed knowledge of how atoms behave. It has only been possible to build equipment like this since our understanding of physics extended to what happens inside atoms.

Scientists are experimenting with attaching anti-cancer drugs to tiny iron particles, then drawing them with a magnetic field to the site of the cancer. The idea came from studying bacteria that produce their own magnetic particles.

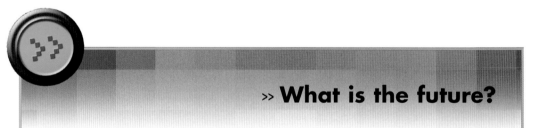

>> What is the future?

Lasers could soon be used to help with skin grafts. At the moment, skin being grafted over an injury is fastened with staples, stitches, or glue. But a dye used in eye operations acts like glue if treated with strong light. After experiments on pig skin, researchers found that the dye can be used to glue grafted skin in place if blasted with a laser. The laser heats the skin only slightly above body heat, so does no damage.

Data from an MRI scan produces a map of the inside of the body when manipulated by computer.

Any questions?

There are few ethical issues surrounding the use of super-beams, but there are questions about safety. When radiation and X-rays were first used, people were not aware of the dangers. We now know that they can damage healthy tissue in the body, and we use them more carefully. Scientists believe that the other scanning techniques commonly used are safe. Ultrasound has been used for a long time, MRI for less time, but no ill effects have been noticed. It is always possible that effects will show up many years after exposure to ultrasound, magnetism, or lasers.

New parts for old

Transplants – replacing a diseased or damaged organ with one from a donor – save thousands of lives each year. But they may be a first step to medical techniques in the future that will not require organs from other people.

Back to basics

A transplant involves taking an organ from one person, usually a person who has died, and putting it into another person whose own organ does not work properly. Many different parts of the body can be transplanted, including hearts, lungs, livers, kidneys, even parts of the eye.

People dreamed of using parts from dead bodies long before we could really do it. Mary Wollstonecraft Shelley wrote the novel *Frankenstein* in 1816.

Landmarks in time	**c. 400 BC** Indian surgeons carry out skin grafts to reconstruct noses and earlobes	**c. 1668** Bone from a dog's skull used to repair a man's skull	**1905** A rabbit kidney is transplanted into a patient with kidney failure, but the patient dies after two weeks.	**1906** First transplant of the cornea (part of the eye) to restore vision, partially successful.

✂ Make the connection

Frenchman Alexis Carrel first learnt about the use of very fine needles and thread in embroidery from his mother. When the president of France was stabbed in 1894, he died because surgeons could not stitch a blood vessel back together. Inspired to improve surgical stitching techniques, Carrel went to one of the finest embroiderers in France to learn about stitching. Already a surgeon, he practised first on paper, then on animal blood vessels to perfect techniques for reconnecting the ends of cut blood vessels. His work made transplants possible.

In 1905, Carrel transplanted a puppy's kidney into a dog. It worked for several hours. By 1908, he had a dog that had lived 17 months after a transplant. Working with Charles Guthrie, he carried out several unsuccessful kidney and **thyroid** transplants in humans and began to study why organs are rejected by the body.

In 1912, Carrel grew heart muscle from a chick embryo in his laboratory. This was the first time living tissue was grown successfully outside the body. He kept it growing for twenty years. On 17 January every year, his team sang "Happy Birthday" to the chicken tissue!

The aviator Charles Lindbergh was prompted by an illness suffered by a family member to design a pump that could keep blood flowing through an organ artificially. Lindbergh built a pump from Perspex, and in 1935, Carrel used the pump to keep a thyroid gland from a cat operational. This meant that transplanting organs from dead people was possible, though it was not made to work until the 1960s.

1952	**1954** First	**1956** First	**1967** First	**1981** First
First kidney transplant from a corpse. The patient died after 22 days.	successful kidney transplant from live donor. The patient lived eight years.	successful bone-marrow transplant	successful heart transplant	successful transplant involving more than one organ (heart and lungs)

It has taken a long time for transplants to become safe and usually successful. The human body is good at identifying foreign material and using the immune system to reject it. This means that transplanted organs are attacked by the patient's body. Doctors have to use special **anti-rejection drugs** to prevent this and give the patient's body time to accept the new organ.

A successful transplant involves careful surgery so that the nerves and blood supply to the new organ are connected properly. Connecting blood vessels is a delicate operation that has been made much easier by modern technology. Clips and stitches are used, but these must dissolve in the body so that the patient does not need another operation to remove them.

Here and now

Many people who once would have died, or had to depend on machines for their whole life, are given a second chance by a transplant operation.

Healthy people register as possible donors. If they die in an accident, or some other way that means they have healthy organs, parts for transplant are removed soon after death. These are kept cool and healthy until they can be put into a person who needs a transplant.

Some body parts can be given by a living donor. People have two kidneys, but need only one to survive, so some people have successfully donated a kidney to help a relative. Bone-marrow transplants from living donors are common, and lungs have also been shared between a living donor and a transplant patient. Individual lobes (sections) of the liver can also be transplanted; this technique can be used to give a child a new liver from part of an adult organ.

Ideas in action

Most of the early transplants were of kidneys and thyroid glands, but now many other organs are transplanted. One of the most complicated transplants is of the heart, or heart and lungs together.

Organs for transplant, such as this heart valve, are sealed in sterile containers and kept cool while transported to where they will be used.

Heart to heart

The first successful heart transplant was carried out by the South African doctor Christiaan Barnard in 1967. The patient survived only 18 days, but it was long enough to prove that the technique could succeed. Over the coming years scientists worked to refine the technique. The development of more effective anti-rejection drugs made an important contribution to the success of later operations. More than 60,000 heart transplants have been carried out.

Fewer hearts become available for transplant than are needed. Scientists have tried using hearts from other animals and building a completely artificial heart. Only a handful of patients with artificial hearts survive. The procedure is only a few years old, and it is too early to say how successful it will be in the long term.

One day, we may farm animals for transplant organs and tissues in the same way that they are now farmed for meat.

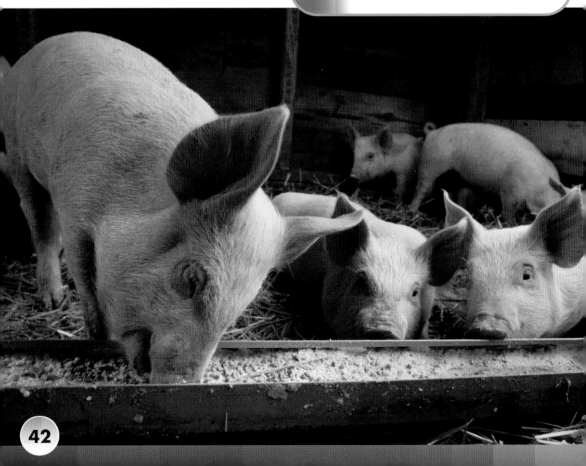

An eye for an eye?

Some transplants are not essential for someone's survival but will make their life easier or more pleasant. As transplant surgery has become more common and more successful, surgeons are willing to use transplants in conditions that do not threaten the patient's life. We can now transplant lots of body parts, such as the larynx (voicebox), womb, jawbone, tongue, and even hands.

>> What is the future?

Could we one day use organs from other animals for transplants? It could offer a way around the shortage of donor organs, but raises other possible problems.

Scientists have experimented with using body parts from animals for many years. As early as the 17th century, surgeons tried to use bone from a dog's skull to mend a human skull. In the early 20th century, several surgeons tried to connect animal kidneys to people's blood supplies (though without implanting them in the body). These early attempts failed. Experiments continued throughout the century with different animals and organs and different methods of connecting or transplanting. The first to show any real promise was a transplant in 1995 of pig embryonic stem cells to help a man with Parkinson's disease, a condition that damages the brain.

Transplants from animals face particular problems of rejection. Researchers are trying to overcome this by creating genetically modified animals – often pigs – which will not produce proteins that the human body rejects.

For many years doctors have discussed the possibility of a face transplant for patients with very severe damage or deformity. Transplants involving skin are amongst the most difficult, with the most severe rejection problems. Scientists have developed very strong anti-rejection drugs and hope they may be able to achieve a face transplant. Permission to carry out a face transplant was given to a hospital in the USA in 2004, though it may take some time to find a suitable donor and patient.

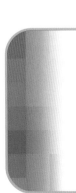

Many people worry that our identities are so bound up in how our faces look that such a transplant could cause real problems for the patient – and for relatives of the donor, who may see someone who looks like their dead relative walking around.

>> What is the future?

There will never be as many organs available for transplant as we need, so scientists are looking at other possibilities.

One solution may be to grow new organs from stem cells. Although growing a single kind of body tissue or cell from stem cells is likely to work soon, growing whole organs is harder as an organ contains many different types of tissue and different structures.

At the same time as research into transplants continues, other developments in artificial organs and tissues may reduce the need for transplants. Artificial organs that will not be rejected would be a better option in many cases. The challenge is to make organs that will work for the rest of the patient's life so that further operations are not needed to mend or replace the new part.

Any questions?

As there is such a shortfall in the supply of donated organs, some people think that we ought to have to opt out of donating our organs if we die, rather than opting in. This would mean that people's organs would be used unless they had previously said they did not want to give them. It would increase the number of organs available, but is it right to take organs without specific permission?

Some people think we should not take transplant organs from animals. They are concerned that our view of ourselves as human might change if we knew we had animal body parts. However, the main barrier to transplants between people and animals is the possibility of some animal infections and diseases affecting people.

Superbugs and superdrugs

People have battled disease for thousands of years. We have made huge progress, but some diseases have developed more dangerous forms that our treatments cannot deal with.

Back to basics

Most illnesses are caused by bacteria or **viruses**. Bacteria are tiny organisms that we often call germs. They are all around us. They usually only make us ill if we are weakened by illness or stress, or if a strain we are not used to turns up. Bacteria are usually killed by **antibiotics**.

Viruses are little more than a strand of DNA. If they get into a cell, they can reproduce and make us ill. They cannot be killed by antibiotics or similar drugs because they are not alive in the same way.

We guard against many illnesses with **vaccinations**. A vaccination gives your body a small dose of a weakened or dead virus or bacterium. Your immune system learns from this how to fight the disease. If you are later exposed to the illness, your immune system can protect you.

✂ Make the connection

The first antibiotic, penicillin, was discovered accidentally by Alexander Fleming in 1928. He was growing a bacterium, *Staphylococcus*, which causes sore throats. His culture became contaminated by a blue/green mould, and he noticed that where the mould was, the bacteria did not grow. He grew the mould and experimented with it, finding that it killed several types of bacteria. Antibiotics were not properly developed for medical use until 1939.

Landmarks in time	**1796** Edward Jenner develops **smallpox** vaccine	**1869** Joseph Lister first uses carbolic acid spray as an **antiseptic** during operations	**1928** Discovery of penicillin, the first antibiotic, by Alexander Fleming	**1980** Smallpox wiped out by a worldwide vaccination programme

In recent years, new diseases have emerged that are very hard to treat. Some are caused by bacteria that our antibiotics cannot kill. Others are caused by viruses we cannot fight.

Here and now

Since the discovery of penicillin, we have developed many more antibiotics that can treat a huge range of infections. Now, many diseases that once killed people are easily cured with antibiotics.

The MRSA bacterium is resistant to many antibiotics and is a serious threat to weakened patients in many hospitals.

Antibiotics are now widely used, not only in human patients but even in the farm animals that produce our milk, meat, and eggs. As a result, some bacteria have adapted so that our antibiotics no longer kill them. Dangerous new strains of disease have appeared that are very difficult to treat. Some can be treated with a mixture of strong antibiotics, but others do not even respond to this.

Combating viruses still depends largely on vaccination to prevent disease, and on boosting the body's own defence system if infection occurs.

Vaccination has wiped out smallpox completely. The virus is kept only in two laboratories, for research purposes. Doctors hope that **polio** will be the next disease to be completely wiped out. We are almost there, but it will take a few more years before it is gone and we are confident that it will not return.

In developed countries, most children are vaccinated against many of the diseases that killed large numbers of people in the past, such as **diphtheria** and **tuberculosis** (TB). As the diseases disappear, though, some countries are giving up the vaccines, and some people choose not to have their children vaccinated. A strain of TB

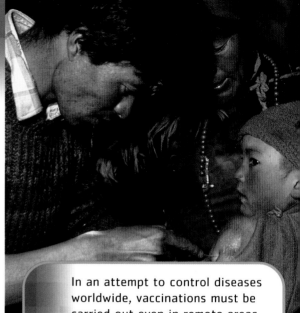

In an attempt to control diseases worldwide, vaccinations must be carried out even in remote areas.

resistant to antibiotics has now appeared in some parts of the world. It is spreading in places where people are not always vaccinated against it, including the UK. One in seven new cases of TB is resistant to treatment.

>< Make the connection

Edward Jenner (1749–1823) was a country doctor. In his time, smallpox was a common and deadly disease. Jenner heard that milkmaids, who frequently caught cowpox, could not get smallpox. He decided that having cowpox must protect them. He took some pus from a cowpox sufferer and injected it into a young boy. He then deliberately injected the boy with smallpox but the boy was protected and the disease did not develop. Jenner had discovered vaccination and his smallpox vaccine became extremely popular.

Vaccinations for other diseases came later, based on the principles of Jenner's work. We now understand how vaccination works with the body's immune system, but Jenner did not know this.

Ideas in action

New diseases are emerging all the time, and some of these offer a tough challenge to modern medicine.

Battling new diseases

Ebola fever first appeared in Africa in 1976. It causes fever, diarrhoea, vomiting, and internal bleeding. Most of the people who catch it die. Ebola fever is caused by a virus. There is no cure for it and no vaccination against it.

HIV destroys the immune system and leads to **AIDS**. It was first identified in 1981 and is now common around the world.

Victims die of other infections, which their bodies cannot fight. There is no cure for HIV, but development of AIDS can be delayed by treatment with drugs to boost the immune system to help keep other infections at bay.

SARS is a respiratory disease. It emerged in the Far East in 2002. A new form of flu, called bird flu, also appeared in the Far East in 1997 and 2003. Originally it could be caught only from birds, but in 2004 a woman apparently caught it from her daughter. Either of these illnesses could become a dangerous, worldwide **epidemic** because flu viruses are difficult to treat and spread very easily.

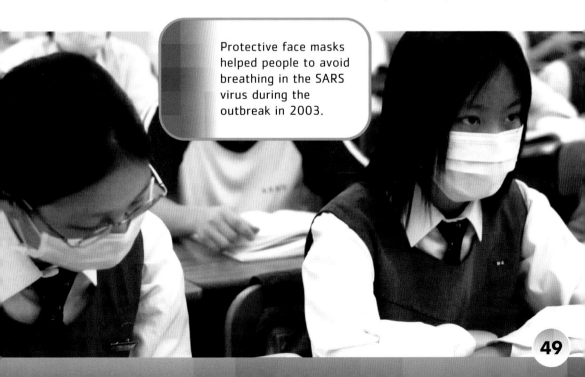

Protective face masks helped people to avoid breathing in the SARS virus during the outbreak in 2003.

Taking care

As we cannot cure these illnesses, health professionals work to prevent them spreading. People who have the diseases are isolated so that they do not infect other people. They are kept in clean conditions to give their immune systems the best chance of combating the disease. The medical staff who care for the patients wear protective clothing, gloves, and masks.

A new epidemic of a disease resistant to treatment is a very frightening prospect. To try to avoid it, researchers use computer models of diseases and epidemics. They work with information about how easily a disease spreads from one person to another, and how many people who get the disease die of it.

Using this information, they can model possible epidemics. They can then decide on suitable precautions such as **quarantine** or preventing international travel.

The hospital superbug

MRSA is an infection that patients in hospital sometimes pick up when they are weakened by operations or illness. It is very hard to treat, and is sometimes fatal. Although it is caused by bacteria, it is resistant to most antibiotics. The UK has the worst MRSA infection rate in Europe, with 7,700 cases in the year 2003/4.

Doctors fear that a version called VRSA, resistant to even our very strongest drugs, could be just around the corner.

✂ Make the connection

Joseph Lister (1827–1912), a surgeon in Scotland, was disturbed by how many patients' wounds became infected. In 1865, he found that spraying carbolic acid onto surgical tools and dressings, and into the air during operations, greatly reduced infections. He had discovered antiseptics. An antiseptic kills the bacteria that cause infections in wounds. By 1869, the number of patients who died after operations carried out by Lister had dropped from 45% to 15%.

Scientists exploring the seabed have found a new type of bacterium that acts as an antibiotic to treat MRSA. Because the new antibiotic is unrelated to any others, MRSA is not resistant to the new drug (called abyssomicin). It may take ten years to turn this discovery into a treatment that can be used in hospitals. Researchers hope that the seabed, which has been little explored so far, may yield many more possibilities for new treatments.

Other new drugs are being developed from crocodile blood and the slime found on the skin of fish!

At a deep sea vent, steam and gases from deep within the Earth burst through the sea bed. Rich in minerals, vents provide a unique habitat supporting many unfamiliar forms of life.

Preventing infection

The huge advances made in public health in the late 1800s came about because doctors realized that dirty conditions encouraged infection and spread disease.

Modern hospitals try to use **aseptic** procedures. Aseptic conditions are even cleaner than antiseptic conditions. It means no bacteria at all should survive to attack patients. It is our best defence against MRSA.

Targeted drugs for cancer interfere with the way a particular cancer is growing, working at a molecular level. Several targeted drugs are being tested on animals at the moment, and some are already in clinical trials on people. They will reduce the unpleasant side effects of treatment, as they will affect only the cancer cells.

As we find out more about our own genes and the genetic make-up of the diseases we are fighting, scientists hope to develop medicines that will work very precisely with particular diseases and even for particular people. The dose or the ingredients of medicines may be adapted to each patient's own genetic profile. There would be fewer side effects, and treatment should be more effective.

Any questions?

Smallpox has been wiped out in the world at large, so hospitals do not need to keep treatments for it, but samples remain for research. Some people think that this is a dangerous situation. What would we do if a terrorist stole or manufactured smallpox? What if a slightly different strain of smallpox emerged? Is it right, or wise, to wipe out a disease, or to keep samples of it for experimentation?

Vaccination can put an end to a disease if everyone is vaccinated. It may soon happen with polio. But not everyone wants to be vaccinated.

In the UK, many parents have refused to have their children vaccinated against mumps, measles, and rubella using the so-called triple vaccine (MMR). They believe the vaccine may occasionally have harmed children. As a result of reduced vaccination, measles has increased in the UK. Measles can only be kept at bay if most people are vaccinated. Is it fair for some people to depend on the immunity of a group but not accept the vaccine? Or should they be forced to have it?

Surgical procedures could one day be carried out by tiny nanorobots put inside the body.

Into the future

Medical advances offer us huge potential to save lives and improve the quality of life. At the same time, further challenges are presented by our changing lives and environments, and further possibilities are opened up as we discover more about our bodies and how they work. There will always be new questions and problems to address, and new avenues for medical scientists to explore.

Glossary

AIDS acquired immuno deficiency syndrome: fatal disease caused by the retrovirus HIV (See also HIV)

anaesthetic a drug or gas that causes a loss of sensitivity to pain

antibiotic treatment for illness or infection caused by bacteria

anti-rejection drug drug to prevent the body rejecting transplanted organs

antiseptic chemical used to prevent infection

aseptic completely clean

bacterium/bacteria microscopic single-cell organism that can cause disease

biotechnology industry that works with natural organisms to make something that people want

bone marrow material in the centre of bones where blood cells are made

cancerous relating to or having cancer

cauterize seal off the ends of blood vessels to stop bleeding

chromosome strand of DNA that carries genetic information

clinical trial test of treatment on human patients

clone exact genetic copy of an organism

computer modelling using a computer to work out how something will behave or to make a copy of something

control group group of patients who are not given a treatment being tested

CT scan computed tomography scan: scan that builds a 3-D image of the inside of the body.

culture medium jelly-like substance on which bacteria and other micro-organisms are grown in a laboratory

diabetes condition in which the body cannot regulate the sugar in the blood properly

diagnostic finding out what is wrong with someone

diphtheria disease that causes serious inflammation of the throat and can be fatal

DNA deoxyribonucleic acid, chemical of which chromosomes are made

donor someone who gives something, such as an organ or blood

embryo unborn baby in the first eight weeks of life

epidemic an outbreak of a disease, that spreads rapidly, afflicting many people

fertility treatment treatment to enable someone to have children

fluorescent giving off light

foetus unborn baby more than eight weeks old.

gene portion of a chromosome holding genetic information about a characteristic or feature

genetic engineering altering genes or genetic material, usually by processes in the laboratory

genetics study of or working with genes

graft a living material, such as skin, that is removed and placed on another body or on another part of the same body

heredity the passing of characteristics from parent to offspring

HIV condition in which the immune system is damaged and the patient falls ill with secondary infections

immune system the body's defence mechanism to help it fight disease

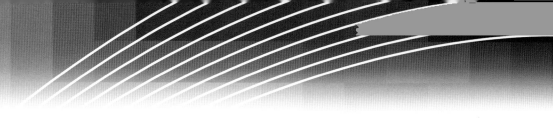

insulin hormone which controls the passing of sugar into the blood

IVF in vitro fertilization: process for fertilizing a human egg outside the body, usually as part of fertility treatment

keyhole surgery surgery carried out through a very small cut in the body

life-support system system of computers and machinery that helps to keep very sick hospital patients alive

MRI scan magnetic resonance imaging scan: scan that builds up an image of the inside of the body by measuring the effect

mutation change in genetic make-up of cells while dividing

nanotechnology very small-scale engineering

nucleus centre of a cell, containing the genetic material

pacemaker implanted machine to regulate the heartbeat

Parkinson's disease disease that slowly destroys the nervous system

placebo pill or medicine which has no physical effect

polio infection affecting the nerve cells in the spinal cord

prototype first form of something new, made before it is produced in large numbers

quarantine period of isolation to prevent the spread of disease

radiation energy that is transmitted as invisible rays

radioactive substance that emits energy at a steady rate

SARS severe acute respiratory syndrome: life-threatening disease of the lungs

side effects unwanted effects of a treatment

smallpox disease which causes painful spots and fever, often fatal

stem cell cell that can produce cells of different types

thyroid gland in the neck which produces a hormone to regulate growth

tissue bodily material made up of cells;

transfusion providing blood or other fluid from another person

transplant take living tissue or an organ and put it in another part of the body or in another body

tuberculosis serious disease that affects the lungs and is often fatal

tumour a mass of extra tissue that grows in or on the body.

ultrasound very high-pitched sound; echoes from ultrasound are used to produce scan images

vaccination treatment with a small dose of a disease in order to build resistance to the disease and prevent infection with it

virus strand of DNA that can change a cell and cause disease

Further resources

Horrible Science: Deadly Diseases, Nick Arnold, Scholastic, 2000

Horrible Science: Microscopic Monsters. Nick Arnold, Scholastic, 2004

Tomorrow's Science: Genetic Engineering, Anne Rooney, Chrysalis, 2003

Tomorrow's Science: Medicine Now, Anne Rooney, Chrysalis, 2003

Index